How to Get Rid of Back Fat

By

Kimberly Peters

For

26Ways.com

Disclaimer

This publication is designed and intended to be used as an educational resource only and not as a definitive action plan for any one specific or individual treatment plan. We are not doctors nor do we represent ourselves as such. You should always consult with your doctor or other medical professional before undergoing any kind of weight or fat loss program. Depending on the health of the individual, some or all of the information contained in this publication may or may not be relevant or appropriate. Your doctor or other medical professional should be the one making the determination of what is right for you. The writers, publishers and sellers of this book assume no responsibility for the use or application of any or all parts of this book. The reader assumes total responsibility for deciding which content, if any, are appropriate for their own health and situation.

Contents

Introduction

If you are reading this book, then I assume that you have an issue with back fat. Either you purchased this book for yourself or someone bought it for you or gave it to you. If that is the case, then before you get started take a moment to smack them in the head for being so insensitive! After you got that out of the way, we can start making some progress.

There are several reasons why we get fat on any part of our body and most of those reasons are the same when it comes to back fat. Contrary to what you might think, there are no foods that have "go directly to the back upon entering the body" in their DNA! When the body creates fat it sends it to wherever it is needed or where it can be stored. Fortunately or unfortunately for us, the back is one of those places.

As we go through the book we will discuss some of the reasons why some of us might have more problem with fat than others and what we can do about it.

It doesn't do us any good to hate those people who mare skinny and have low body fat.

They are either incredibly fortunate or work really hard at keeping fat off. We need to concern ourselves only with our own bodies and no one else's.

Before we get started, I want to first talk about health for a moment. Our health is far more important to us than the way we look in a bathing suit or a tight pair of pants or dresses. Appearance is important as everyone wants to look good both to themselves and others but our individual health is much more important.

We mention this because there are all kinds of fad diets and products designed to help you lose weight. Some of these products might work but a lot of them just make your wallets lighter while doing nothing for you. But the greater danger comes from trying to lose weight or reduce fat too quickly or in any unhealthy manner.

Because of this, I strongly advise anyone who is trying to lose weight or change their body style or appearance in any way to at least consult with their doctor before doing anything. This is especially true for anyone with any kind of health issues or disease such as diabetes, high blood pressure or any other disease.

When it comes to exercise, also be aware that too much can be just as bad, sometimes even worse, than not enough. It is very easy to get carried away and try to do too much too soon.

You can strain or tear muscles and do other damage to your body if you try to exceed what is safe for you. There are many factors that go into designing the proper weight training or workout. Because of this, you might wish to consider hiring a personal trainer if only to help you get started. They can evaluate you and set up a proper exercise program for you and show you the proper way to use the equipment and the correct form to use when doing the exercises.

Your goals should not be on getting to the goal as quickly as possible unless there is a health reason to do so. Instead your goal should be to design a program that is manageable and that you will be able to stick with for an extended period of time. People who are able to do that are almost always much more successful and tend to achieve their goals more easily than those who try to go through a crash program designed only for quick results.

Last, but certainly not least, your ultimate goal should include making the changes you need to lose the fat but also adopt a lifestyle that will allow those changes to stay in place for a long period of time. If we make temporary changes and then go back to what we were doing that caused the problem in the first place, the fat and weight will come right back and we will have to start all over again.

The great news is that almost everyone will be able to get rid of their back fat and look good in whatever clothes they want. The bad news is that there is no magic pill or product that will get you there overnight with little or no effort. Those are marketing ploys designed to get you to part with your hard earned money.

But if you want to make meaningful changes and you want a healthy and responsibly way of going about it, then turn the page and start reading.

The Myth of Spot Fat Reduction

We often say that the hot fudge sundae that we just ate for dessert is going straight to our hips or stomach. But the fact is, it goes to those places plus a whole lot of other places as well. Excess calories do not just go to our waist. They go to our face, our chin, thighs and also to our back.

The same also goes for getting rid of fat and losing weight. To the best of my knowledge there are no exercises that will burn off calories in just one particular area. You rarely see a skinny man or woman with 12 chins and chubby cheeks because as we lose weight and burn off calories, we take fat from all over our body to provide those calories.

Now that doesn't mean that you don't notice the change more in certain areas because we had more fat cells in that particular area.

For example if you go on a diet or start exercising you will see and feel a difference around your waist because that is where most of our excess fat usually is located. So you will see that your pants are less tight or getting loose and you might feel better or different as well.

But at the same time you are noticing the stomach getting smaller there are also changes going on with your face, thighs and other areas. But since there are less fat cells in those areas the changes are much less noticeable. But in a few weeks or months you will look in the mirror and notice that you have one less chin or more definition in your facial features.

The good part of this is as you try to reduce the area of back fat that you have you will also be improving other areas of your body as well. So you get additional benefits from your efforts. But the bad part of this is that if you have 5 pounds of back fat to get rid of you might have to lose 10-15 pound of other fat to get rid of, or at least reduce, your back fat.

The other way we can get rid of the appearance of fat in a certain area is by targeting that area with exercises designed to strengthen and build muscle in that area. This helps build definition and firm up areas that once were flabby and not well defined. So the same amount of fat might still be there but building muscle helps mask it and make the entire overall area look and feel better.

Because of this it is usually better to combine fat reduction with building and toning muscle. This helps us get better results in less time. Muscle building and strengthening is also important because as we build muscle we help tighten up areas that might get flabby or saggy as we lose weight. Plus, muscle requires more calories to sustain so the more muscle we have the more calories we will burn every day and that will help us lose more fat or at least keep that fat off.

So let's forget about just targeting one area of our body and instead create a plan that addresses not only our back fat but our entire body. We want to look better, feel better and live healthier. We should think about losing our back fat as an added bonus so as we live longer and healthier we will also look better as well.

So as we move forward and design our plan and approach, let's take our entire body into consideration so we can tackle everything at once to get the best results in the least amount of time.

And let's always remember to do so in a healthy and responsible way so that we not only look better but that we also feel better and live healthier all at the same time. After all, what's the point of looking better if we don't feel better at the same time?

Metabolism and Age Factors

Have you ever noticed how some people have to be careful and watch everything they eat or they gain weight? Have you also known people who can eat 15 meals a day and have soda and ice cream with each one and never gain a darned ounce? I'm not sure which one you are like but I think I can say you are probably in the first group if you have a problem with back fat.

Some of us are just born with genetics that give us lean bodies no matter what we eat. We are just born with a body that has a high metabolism and a body structure that does not make it easy for fat to gain a stronghold in your body. Having a high metabolism means that our bodies burn more calories throughout the day and do not allow calories to turn them into fat very easily.

It has also been said that all out bodies have a certain number of fat storage cells and this also plays a role in how easy it is to gain weight and where that weight is carried on the body. The theory is that skinny people have fewer fat storage cells while heavier people have more of these cells. In fact liposuction is a process where certain fat cells are removed from the body causing those parts of the body to look thinner and more sculpted immediately.

While metabolism is built into our own genetics, it is possible to improve our metabolism by proper diet and exercise. If we eat the right healthy foods, and get some exercise on a regular basis we can increase our metabolism. Which means that not only are we ingesting fewer calories in the foods we eat, we are also burning more through exercise and an increased metabolism. The result is that we lose weight easier and faster as long as we keep up eating healthy and exercising.

One other factor when it comes to getting rid of fat and losing weight is the role our age plays in the process. Even though we can change the foods we eat and increase the amount of exercise we get, the one thing we cannot control or work on is how old we are.

As we age things in our bodies change. Where we were once thin or rock solid we know have a love handle or two and a bit of a belly. We might also weigh the same but that weight has distributed itself around our bodies differently. It is amazing how we might have weighed the same amount in college as we do now but now the weight is carried much differently on our frames.

Though no two people are exactly alike, one generalization can often be made when it comes to weight, body composition and age.

That generalization is that as we get older it will require more work and a stricter diet to even keep our bodies in their current condition. It also likely means that we will have to eat less to keep from gaining weight and adding fat as well. In other words the days of scarfing down a half pound burger and fries with friends at 10 0'clock at night are long over!

As we get older muscle tone and the overall amount of muscle in our bodies tends to drop as well. Since muscle requires more calories each day the more muscle we have the easier it is to lose weight and keep the fat off. But as we age our fat percentage goes up and our muscle mass tends to go down.

All this is because as we get older our metabolism changes as well. We rarely get the same amount of exercise as we did when we were younger and our lifestyle often become more sedentary and less strenuous as well.

All this results in our metabolism slowing down and along with it the number of calories we burn doing the same every day activities.

So don't feel bad if it takes you longer to get the results you are looking for. As we age our bodies help make things get a little more difficult every year. But if we remain patient and committed to the process we can still get the success we want as long as our expectations are reasonable.

In other words, if you are in your 50's don't expect a defined and well-toned body of a 20-year old because it ain't gonna happen. You can get close and you can look younger because you are healthier but you will still have the body and skin of a 50 year old when you are 50 and that is going to help determine how much effort is going to be required to get the right results.

Hormones and Insulin Resistance

Sometimes how our bodies react to our everyday lives can have a profound impact on how we look as well. Two factors we also have to consider in addition to metabolism and age are hormone levels and insulin resistance. Both of these have a significant impact on how our body's process sugars and create or store fat.

Hormones such as cortisol tell the body to store fat. They cause the brain to send messages to the body that it needs to create and store fat for possible use for the future. When this happens we gain weight in the form of fat and that fat will settle throughout the body including around the waist and on the back.

Since we strongly suggested in the beginning of this book that you consult with your doctor before going on any kind of weight loss or exercise regimen, this might be a good time to discuss health related issues including hormone levels if you feel that you are gaining weight far too easily or that your diet is much too restrictive when you need to either lose weight or stay at your current weight.

Your doctor might suggest a blood test to check for various hormone levels to make sure that all are within the normal range. If one of more are not, he or she might prescribe medication to help your body create normal hormone levels. This is important because if hormones are the reason for your weight gain, it might be extremely difficult, if not impossible to make the changes you want without medical help.

Insulin resistance refers to how efficiently the body uses and responds to insulin levels within the body. People with high insulin resistance have cells in their body that are resistant to the effects of insulin in the bloodstream. Though commonly thought of as a diabetic problem, it can affect non-diabetics as well although at a smaller level.

Insulin resistance is associated with obesity, especially when there is significant fat around the abdominal area as well as high blood pressure and high cholesterol.

Since all of those problems represent potentially serious medical conditions, if you have any of those conditions you should see your doctor and allow him to create a plan for you to follow to lose the weight you wish to lose.

We would also like to point out that sometimes certain medical conditions such as high blood pressure, and sometimes diabetes will provide no symptoms or such mild symptoms that they are easily overlooked or attributed to something else. The result is that we allow these conditions to go untreated and undiagnosed for longer periods of time. During this time damage may be occurring to the body which may or may not be permanent. So be sure to have regular check-ups and have blood work done whenever your doctor suggests it. This is the best way to stay healthy and minimize the effects and damage caused by any health related problem in your body.

Getting back to losing weight and back fat, not resolving potential hormone and insulin resistance issues will make it that much harder for you to accomplish your goals. You will have to work much harder, for a longer period of time in order to achieve your goals. So it makes sense to make sure you are healthy and that any potential problems are either eliminated or treated so you can not only look good but feel good and live longer as well.

Overall Body Fat

Like we said before, back fat is just one area of fat that is in your body. So it is important to deal with the entire body and not just one area. Exercises that target just the back might be effective in helping that one area but other exercises that deal with aerobic and cardio activity will give you better overall results than just exercises that target the back.

Another problem with losing fat sometimes is that we do not know when we are making progress. With weight loss it is easy because we can hop on the scale and see our weight on the dial or readout. If we weighed less than what we weighed a few days ago then our efforts are paying off. If we weight the same or more, then we know we have to either do more or eat less. A scale is direct feedback on our progress or lack of and it helps us remain motivated or lets us know when additional changes are needed.

When it comes to fat, however, the issue gets a little trickier. We can lose fat without seeing a significant change in weight. In some cases, as we exercise and build muscle, we might even weigh a bit more even though we lost fat. This is because fat weighs less than muscle so when we lose fat and increase muscle, we actually gain weight!

When there is significant fat in a couple of areas, mostly the abdomen, we can tell we are losing fat by noticing that our pants or other clothes are fitting better or getting looser. We might also notice that we are going in a notch or two on our belts as well. All of these are physical changes that are easy to notice.

But when it comes to the back, or other areas of the body where fat is stored in lesser quantities, this can become a problem when it comes to measuring our success or lack of. In these cases we need something else to help us accomplish our goals and lose our fat.

Fortunately there are products available to us that make measuring body fat easier than it ever has been. We usually were told to try and pinch around our waist and see how much we were able to pinch. That would be an indication of the presence of excess fat. But the problem with that approach was that it was hugely inaccurate and sometimes very misleading. It relied on a subjective look that was subject to a wide degree of interpretation and guesswork.

Plus, it was difficult, if not impossible to measure a change of just a pound or two of fat. The only advantage of this method was that it was free. It wasn't accurate but it didn't cost us anything either.

But today we can purchase home scales that measure body fat and BMI (Body Mass Index) so that we can see how much fat we really have in our bodies at any given time. These scales are not expensive and give us a great way to see exactly what is happening with the fat in our bodies. They are just slightly more expensive than a regular digital scale. Sometimes the big box stores or Amazon have them on sales and you can get one at a really great price.

If you can gain access to a scale that can measure body fat, then use it once a week and keep a record of your progress or lack of. This will enable you to see what is working for you and what is not. It is nice to have actual accurate data on which to measure progress.

Use this in conjunction with a weight journal and your overall feeling of how your clothes fit and how you physically feel. Using these three methods of tracking fat loss will help you understand how well you are doing and how your body is responding.

When it comes to back fat the importance of a scale is even more important because you cannot easily see back fat except when you are wearing clothes. While you can easily grab your waist or "love handles" and see how you are doing it is not that easy to do the same with fat in areas you cannot reach. Plus, changes in the amount of back fat are going to be subtle and only noticeable gradually over time so you might get discouraged without some accurate data.

Think of losing back fat as a part of losing fat over your entire body. Fat lost in your abdomen also means that some fat was also lost in or around your back and legs as well. So don't obsess with your back, concentrate on an entire body action plan. You will find you get better results in less time if you approach your goal in that manner.

Increasing Cardio

When it comes to exercise, we receive two primary benefits from exercise. The first is health as exercise helps our bodies stay in better condition and better able to handle the everyday stress and strain of life as well as being able to defend itself against disease and infection. The second benefit is that it helps us either stay at a normal and healthy weight or allows us to reduce our weight.

When it comes to weight reduction, exercise helps us in two ways. Certain types of exercise allows us to burn calories and therefore reduce fat and weight. The other types of exercise help us build muscle and increase strength. Most exercise programs use a combination of the two exercise types to allow us to look better, firm up our bodies while also increasing strength and stamina at the same time.

For the purposes of this book, however, we are going to concentrate on the type of exercise that will help us shed fat and weight and tone up areas of our bodies. That means we are going to have to incorporate a few different type of exercise into our program. The most important type of exercise that we need to increase is cardio.

Cardio exercise refers to the types of exercise that cause our heart rates to rise and get our entire body into exercise mode. General types of exercise might include walking, jogging, running, treadmill, stair master and any other form of exercise that helps us get our heart rate (pulse) into the target area.

Cardio exercise helps us burn and shed fat faster for a few important reasons. Once you understand why cardio is so important and how it works, you will be more eager to get some more cardio into your daily life.

Cardio gets our pulse rate up and that increases the number of calories we burn while exercising. So the result is that whenever we burn more calories we either lose weight or can eat more because we burned more calories during that day. Assuming you are not going to eat more because you exercised, the result will be loss of weight and loss of body fat as well.

But the great thing about cardio exercise is that the body continues to burn more calories per hour for several hours even after you are finished exercising.

So if you do cardio for an hour you will burn more calories per hour for that hour and for several hours afterwards. So the benefit of cardio exercise continue long after the exercising is completed.

One reason this happens is that people who have cardio exercising in their daily routine often benefit from having a higher metabolism as well. This is because our bodies have the unique ability to change how they operate based on the demands we place on them. So if the body knows it is going to have to run every other day it will create a metabolism and body structure better equipped to handle that workload.

In order to get the most benefit from cardio exercise doctors tell us that we must do cardio for at least 30 minutes to get the benefits. If you can do an hour you will do even better but do not overdue it. Talk with your doctor about which forms of cardio exercising is right for you and how long and what intensity is safe for you.

If you are used to cardio exercise that is wonderful. But if you are not, it is best to work into it gradually and not try and go all out at once. If you try and do too much too soon, you might find yourself sore, or even worse, and you might actually do more harm than good. So start slow and gradually work up to what your body is capable of.

The great thing about cardio exercise is that there are cardio exercises for just about everyone. Even people of advanced ages can walk and this also applies to people who are in very poor physical condition. You have heard the expression "You need to walk before you can run" and this is never truer than when it comes to cardio exercise!

Just walking around the block is considered cardio exercise! Start with once around the block at a slow pace and then gradually increase the time and the speed as your body adjusts and is able to handle the higher stress and workload. Some people never get past walking and that is fine. Just get out there and move and get some exercising to get your body into fat-burning mode.

Ask your doctor what your target heart-rate should be for someone your age and in your particular physical condition. Generally speaking the older you are the lower your target rate is going to be. But if your physical condition and health allow, if you can get your heart rate up into the 120 or so range that is good for cardio benefits. But once again I caution you that everyone is different and your doctor should tell you what your target rate should be. Do not allow any book to tell you what is safe for you. There are just too many variables to consider when making that determination.

Circuit Training

So much of body sculpting and toning involves working on the entire body and not just one particular area. Losing body fat is no different. That is why if you have access to it, circuit training can be a real help in creating the type of body you want.

Circuit training usually refers to using a "circuit" of machines that each target a certain part of the body. In a gym you will find machines for arms, legs, abdominals, back, shoulders and just about any part of the body you might need to exercise. The object is to go through all of the machines so that each major muscle group is exercised. The result is burning more calories, exercising more muscles and giving your body better definition and toning.

For those who do not have access to a gym or circuit machine, you can still do exercises that target different parts of the body.

Various exercises like sit-ups, jumping jacks, push-ups and running each target different muscle groups yet require no specialized equipment or investment.

The advantage of using machines is that you are exercising in a more controlled environment where the entire exercise process is more defined and exact and safer. With machines you can use precise weights and settings so you cannot exceed what is safe for you. These machines also provide safety in that you can stop any time you want, drop a weight bar without injuring yourself and other benefits.

But regardless of whether you use machines or individual exercises, make your doctor aware of what you want to do and get their approval first. They will help you develop a healthy and safe way of getting the exercise you need without placing your body in harm's way.

Yoga

Even though it may look strange and not appear to be difficult or strenuous, Yoga can be a great way to tone your body, get the definition that you need and improve your overall flexibility. For those with certain health or body issues Yoga can also be a great way of getting the exercise you need without the risks or side effects of other exercise.

One advantage of Yoga is that it is low impact. Low impact means there is not very much impact or stress placed on your joints while exercising. People with bad knees or hips, for example, might not be able to run, or even walk because of the impact and jarring that occurs with each step.

Running, for example, has more impact than jogging and jogging has more impact than walking. So if you have issues or problems with your knees, feet, legs or hips, then running might be out while jogging and walking might be OK. Or, you might have to limit yourself to walking only.

Yoga is also good because the positions you use will help you tone specific areas of your body almost without you knowing it! I had shoulder surgery several years ago and could not move my arm out from my side at all without pain. But I realized that after a Yoga class I had almost twice the range as I did before I started! All by just following some basic slow and flowing moves that gently stretched out the muscles in the body.

Yoga also works on the "core" of the body and that is where we get most of our overall strength and stability from. The stronger our core is the better overall condition we find ourselves in.

As far as back fat is concerned, poses such as the "half-moon", "Bow yoga" and the "wheel" target the abdominal and back muscles. This will help you provide tone to the back area as well as reduce overall body fat.

If this sounds like something you might be interested in, I suggest you join a local yoga class and learn some of the basics from a licensed and experienced Yoga instructor. This might be an enjoyable way for you to get exercise as well as reducing your back fat and fat in other areas of the body as well.

Other benefits of Yoga are lowering of blood pressure, stress reduction and improving the body's metabolism and ability to heal and fight infection as well. In other words, there are more benefits to Yoga than just flexibility and weight loss!

Personal Trainers

Sometimes it helps to get someone on our side when it comes to helping us achieve an objective or goal. Getting another person involved also helps us stay committed and focused as well. But when that other person has specific knowledge that can help us even further, that person might be something we really want to consider adding to our team.

Personal trainers are people with specific knowledge of exercise and how it effects the human body. They will talk to you about your goals and objectives and evaluate your individual health and physical condition and develop a healthy and responsible program to help you lose back fat and other fat in your body.

The benefit of having a person trainer is that they help keep you motivated and determined. They are people who will push you further than you are likely to push yourself. They will motivate you, encourage you and make the process easier for you.

In addition, personal trainers, because of their knowledge of exercise and its effects, are usually able to get you better results in less time and also do that in a healthy and responsible manner. That is why so many people use them when they have an important date in the future, such as a wedding or other social event that they want to look good for.

You can use personal trainers in a few different ways.

You can hire a personal trainer to work with you throughout the entire process until you achieve your objective or attain your goals. When used in this manner they will constantly update and tailor your exercises to meet your needs at that particular time. So as you see results they can increase or change exercises to help better results or help you move on to the next level. This is the most intensive and expensive option for most people.

Another option might be to hire a trainer for a few sessions so that they can work on showing you the correct exercises that you should be doing and also the correct form you should be using while doing them. This is important because when doing certain exercises you need to do them correctly in order to get the right benefits from them. In this option the trainer will design a program for you, get you started and then you take it from that point on. You might be able to go back from time to time as you make progress.

This option is less expensive while still giving you access to a trainer to design the workout for you.

The last option is hiring a trainer for the consultation and designing of the program and then taking that information home with you and doing everything on your own. With this option you can get the program designed and then go from there. This option lacks the personal attention and motivation but if money is an object it will allow you to know what you need to do and then do it on your own. This is the least expensive option.

Only you know which option is best for you.

Personally, I find that option two is the best compromise for most people if money is an issue. Scheduling a trainer for a few sessions will not only get your started but will also give you the opportunity to "practice" some of the exercises under their watchful eyes so that they can correct any flaws or issue concerning form, speed and technique.

In some areas you can hire a trainer at a local gym on a per session basis. They will take you around to the various machines and show you how to adjust them, use them and how to perform each exercise. The cost for this is minimal and might help you learn a little bit about what needs to be done and how to go about safely.

Whatever option you choose it will usually include an initial physical evaluation so that you can understand what needs to happen and what areas need your attention. This can come in useful as they might tell you about things you never knew about as far as your own body shape and condition.

Water –A Key Weight Loss Ingredient!

A critical part of ever healthy lifestyle is making sure the body gets all the water it needs before it needs it. Failure to properly hydrate the body can cause all kinds of problems from muscle cramps to kidney problems.

Many people think it is smart to reduce the amount of water because water means weight. They think it is great to lose 4 pounds during a run or walk because that is all sweat and now you weigh 4 pounds less.

Well, I've got news for you! You did not burn 14,000 calories (4 pounds X 3,500 calories) in that walk! You lost water weight due to sweating and exertion. You need to replace that water so your body and continue to provide the chemical actions that go on inside your body.

We also said in a paragraph about that we need to make sure we give our bodies the water they need BEFORE they need it. That means drinking water before you work out and continuing to drink during your exercise and after wards as well. This will allow your body to function properly. I read one doctor say if you wait until you're thirsty, you waited too long!

Our muscles and systems need water to function properly. You cannot expect a dehydrated body to be able to continue to function let alone exercise. Left unaddressed, dehydration can cause passing out and even death!

It has long been said that the average person should drink 6-8 glasses of water every day. This is the figure for average people with average exercise levels. Someone who exercises or sweats a lot needs MORE that those 6-8 glasses each day. They might need 10-12 or more depending on what they do and where they do it.

Let's get one thing very clear right now, though.

When we refer to getting 6-8 glasses of water a day, we mean WATER! We do not count beer or soda or fruit juices or flavored drinks. Water is the very best drink for overall body health. It contains no calories, artificial sweeteners and none of the crap that is in those processed drinks we all drink.

And a word about soda and alcohol too. Alcohol actually dehydrates you as you drink! The more alcohol you drink the more water you need as well. Soda is another drink that actually dehydrates you as you drink it. Soda has a lot of salt in it. It's designed to make you thirsty so you will drink more of it! For every can or either regular or diet soda you drink, you should ADD one glass of water to your daily requirement!

Benefits of Drinking Water

Drinking water has other benefits as well for our weight loss plan. First of all, water has no calories but it takes calories for the body to process it and run it through our digestive systems. So drinking water helps us burn calories and lose weight!

The other important thing water does is help flush toxins and by products from our bodies. This helps keep our bodies clean of these substances and helps it function at a higher level.

How to Get Enough Water

Some people have a hard time getting their 6-8 glasses of water a day. Not because it is difficult but because they just don't think about it or count what they drink.

For those people, the best thing to do is to keep a jug of cold water in the refrigerator and drink from it throughout the day. You might even be right that drinking cold water requires more calories to process but the main reason is that the jug lets you know how close or how far you are away from your 6-8 glasses. If the jug isn't empty, you are not finished yet!

You can substitute water for soda or wine at meals as well. This has a double effect because you should be adding to your 6-8 glasses for the soda and alcohol that you drink throughout the day! So changing to water will help you make your 6-8 glasses go easier and faster.

If you have questions about how much water you should drink every day, be sure to check with your doctor. He or she will be able to give you more information and guidance.

Do Back Exercises

While this is by all means not a complete listing of exercises that target the back and back fat, they are enough to get you started in toning your back and getting rid of your back fat. But before you attempt any of these exercises check with your doctor or medical professional to make sure you are healthy enough to attempt them. Even then, do them safely and with moderation. Too much too soon will not help anyone get to where they need to be!

Exercise One: Go Flying!

Lie on your stomach with your body stretched out and your arms out in front of you. Then, at the same time, lift up your arms and your legs towards the ceiling and hold for 5 seconds. Then relax for a few second and repeat. Do 2-3 sets of 10-15 if you are able. If not, do what you can safely do. If you experience pain at any time, stop.

Exercise Two: Row, Row, Row Your Boat!

If you own a rowing machine then do some rowing to build up your shoulders and strengthen you back muscle to provide definition and toning. If you don't own a rowing machine, or if they don't have one at the gym, then make your own by using an exercise band.

Sit down with your legs straight out in front of you and place one end of the exercise band around your feet. Then while sitting up straight with your arms slightly bent inhale and then exhale as you bring your arm in until your elbows are behind you. Do not move your torso. All movement should be by your arms. Keep all movements slow and controlled with no jerking movements or fast motions. Do a dozen of these if you are able.

Exercise Three: Go for a Swim!

Lying flat on your stomach on a padded mat with your arms and legs straight out, lift your chest up and raise your arms and legs. Then go through "swimming" motions by moving your arms and legs alternately up and down. Go as high up as is comfortable. Continue this exercise for one minute if possible.

Exercise Four: The Bridge

Lay flat on your back on a padded mat or carpet. Then bring your legs up until they are approx. a foot from your pelvis.

Now arch your spine so that you raise your rear end off the mat until your spine is relatively straight. You should now be in a bridge position. Then push one heel into the mat and raise the other leg with the knee still bent. Raise the leg approx. 90 degrees and hold it for a few seconds then lower it and repeat with the other leg. Do this for approx. one minute.

Exercise Five: Don't Be a Dumbbell, Use Them!

Stand upright and then bend over at slightly less than a 90 degree angle. Allow your arms to hand with each hand holding a 5 or 10 pound weight. (Whichever feels better. You can always start with the 5 and move up later.) Then take your arms, bend them at the elbow and bring them up and past your back. Do this for one minute.

Then, in the same basic position, bend your arms at the elbow and move them outwards and hold for a second or two and then return to the normal position. Repeat for one minute. These two exercises will work out back muscles to provide more definition.

Exercise Six: Plank It!

Though this exercise looks simple and easy, once you try it you will see why it is so effective in strengthening your core and back muscles!

Lie on your stomach and then place your arms at roughly your shoulder line and raise your body up until your arms arm straight. This is sort of like a push-up. Now hold that pose with your spine straight. Hold for a minute or two if you can!

If you can do that one then try this variation as well:

From the same position with your arms straight and your spine straight, lift one arm out to the side and then return it in place and repeat with the other arm. Do 10 reps each side.

Exercise Seven: Go for a Swim!

Swimming is one of the best exercises for anyone looking to lose weight or eliminate fat. It is very effective for back fat removal as well because the muscles we use during swimming are the same muscles we need to work on for back fat removal! So not only can we get refreshed by a nice swim in some cool water, we can get exercise and tone those areas where we want to look better.

Lean Out Your Diet

It just makes sense that if you wish to get rid of some of the fat in your body that you cannot continue to put fat into your body at the same time if you expect to get results. That means changing the way we eat and the foods we eat. Otherwise we are just going to have a vicious cycle where we remove fat and then go ahead and put it right back in and replace it.

While this is not a diet book per say, what we eat does have a direct correlation on the amount of fat in our body and how successful we are in removing it. With that in mind, here are a few things to take into consideration when it comes time to decide what we eat and how much of it we do eat:

Portion Size

This is a reason why obesity is a problem in the world today and one of those reasons is portion size.

If you go out to eat or buy a sandwich these days it seems that everyone is trying to make theirs the biggest and best. Everyone is pushing "super-size" and larger sizes of just about everything.

Think about this for a minute: If you go to a fast food place and get a large drink that could be 32-48 ounces of soft drink. That is the same as 3-4 cans of soda! If you were eating that meal at home there is no way you would down 3-4 cans of soda during the meal. Common sense would tell you that you shouldn't do that!

The same thing goes for the food we eat as well. No one goes to the supermarket and buys a pound of chopped meat and gets just two burgers out of it but we don't think twice about getting an 8 or 10 ounce burger at a restaurant! In fact we eat SO much more when we go out it is a miracle that we aren't even larger than most of us already are!

Limit your portion size by either cooking just what you need or just putting enough on your plate for you and keeping the rest off the table. Avoid family style servings where huge platters of food are sitting in front of you on the table. If necessary, use measuring cups to measure out the portion size you want. Very often our eyes deceive us and we wind up eating 2-3 times what we thought we were eating!

Carbohydrates

Carbohydrates are what gives us energy but they also convert extremely easily to sugar and fat as well. That means we should control the amount of breads and starches we eat as well as sweets and anything that is high in carbohydrates. If you are diabetic you understand the role carbs play in controlling blood sugar.

We do need carbs for energy and they play an important role in our nutrition but most of us eat entirely too many carbs in our normal diet. But once you become aware of this it is fairly easy to cut down on carbs while still maintaining a good lifestyle and being able to eat the food we enjoy.

Drinks

Most of us are not aware of the number of calories we consume through beverages every day. Soft drinks can have over 150 calories in just one small can and those gigunda drinks at the fast food store can pack over 600 calories! When you figure that the standard adult diet is around 2,000 calories you can see how dropping 600-800 calories on beverages is not a great idea!

Water is the best hydrator and it is cheap and readily available as well. But diet sodas have the taste and fizz we enjoy without all the sugars and calories.

Beware of fruit juices as well as a lot of them are loaded with sugar and carbs as well! So that orange juice you think is healthy is really a calorie loaded carbohydrate bomb!

Alcohol

Beer and hard liquor is loaded with calories as well. And like soft drinks, those calories can really add up over the course of an evening! And for those of you who think light beer has few calories, there are plenty of fat people sitting on bar stools drinking lite beer!

Have a drink or two and follow them up with water or diet soda for the rest of the evening. An added benefit is that no one has received a ticket for driving under the influence of diet soda!

Lean Meats

Most of us love meat, especially red meat, but if we choose leaner cuts of meat that have less fat, we are doing both our bodies and our waistlines a favor as well. Substituting leaner meats like pork and chicken for red meat will help as well.

As a rule the less fat we put into our body the less fat we will find in those places we don't want to see it!

Read Labels!

On just about any packaged food we purchase these days you will see nutrition labels. These labels are there to help people like you and I choose the healthiest foods when it comes time to prepare a meal. If you stop and take the time to read these labels, you often find that there are big differences between brands and ingredients and the number of calories and carbs!

Since the most successful diets are the ones that are the easiest to follow, it just makes sense to us the information on the labels to make the best choices. This will enable us to keep more of the foods we like in our diets. This way we will stick with them longer and have a better chance of achieving our goals.

Be Colorful!

Sometimes some of the easiest tips are among the most effective! If you cook and eat vegetables that are bright in colors and eat a rainbow of these vegetable then you will have a pretty good chance of eating better than you are now. Your plate should look like a rainbow of colors! And for the real wise guys reading this, jelly beans do not count no matter how colorful they might be!

Be a Clock Watcher!

Sometimes it is not just what we eat but when we eat it that can make all the difference in the world. If we sit down in the evening and eat a bunch of snacks right before bedtime, it results in lowering your metabolism and causing more of those calories to be turned into fat instead of being burned off through normal daily activity.

Try and stop eating and snacking a few hours before bedtime and maybe even get in a little bit of light exercise as well. You will not only sleep better and feel better but you will create less fat and help yourself meet your goals far more easily!

Be Honest With Yourself

No matter what we need to do and how long we have to do it, we will not stand a chance of success if we cannot be honest with ourselves in the process. If we tell ourselves that bag of chips is only one serving even though the bag says it's 4 servings, then we are only kidding ourselves.

The same applies to exercise. If we constantly make excuses for not exercising, we are hurting no one but ourselves. We can always find excuses for not doing those things we don't like and all of that is fine if that is what you really want. But if you want to achieve a goal or hit an objective, then you need to be honest with yourself and do the things you know you need to do. If you cannot do that, then do not get upset with anyone but yourself if you do not achieve your goals.

Setbacks are normal for most of us and there will be times when we eat something we shouldn't of miss exercise to see our favorite TV program and all of that is fine. We are entitled to have a treat or be a little lazy at times. But the important thing is to just get back in the routine and start back up doing the things that we need to do in order to be successful.

Drink More Water

When it comes to losing weight and fat on any part of your body, drinking water is an important part of the process. Water helps hydrate the body and keep it properly functioning during exercise and throughout the day. While many people feel that water weight is to be avoided, the fact remains that drinking more water will help you lose weight and fat faster.

Water helps the body rid itself of toxins and various kinds of waste. Toxins and other by-products leave the body through urine and as they do that, allows the body to function better and more efficiently.

Water weight is temporary and will not lead to you increasing the amount of fat or muscle in the body. So if you drink 10 gallons of water you might weigh more of the scale today but in a day or so you will be back to normal.

Drinking water also causes toe body to burn more calories as well. Though not a tremendous amount of calories, whenever the body has to do anything that requires calories. So processing water into urine so that it can exit the body will require the body to burn more calories.

While the actual amount of water may vary, the average adult requires approx. 8 glasses of water per day or about 64 ounces. This is the minimum amount of water required to keep the body healthy and hydrated. Failure to keep the body properly hydrated and lead to other health related problems.

Lack of water can cause the urine to become more concentrated which often leads to the formation of kidney stones. These can be extremely painful when it comes time to pass them. Staying properly hydrated can protect you from creating kidney stones unless there are other reasons for their formation.

When it comes to weight and fat loss, water is very important. And when we say water we mean water. Sod or beer is not a substitute for water. Soda and beer have a lot of calories while water does not. Even diet soda, which has a very low number of calories, contains a lot of sodium or salt which can cause you to retain water instead of processing it and that will lead to weight gain.

Drink your water throughout the day. Do not go thirsty all day long and then binge drink at night. Keep a water bottle on your desk or beside you at home and drink all day long. As we said, 8 ounces is the minimum. More is perfectly fine as long as you don't mind getting up to go to the bathroom all day!

Get a Massage!

I seriously doubt if I am going to get any arguments from a single reader when it comes to this chapter! That is because we are going to talk about something that will not only make you feel really great all at the same time!

Massages help break down fatty tissue and also help the body break down toxins and make it easier for the body to rid itself of those toxins. All the manual pressure and kneading and stretching helps us stay flexible and healthy.

You don't need a painful or extremely deep massage to reap the benefits either. In fact, there is something to be said about a nice relaxing and stress busting massage! Tell the therapist about any problem areas that you would like them to work on. This could be the back for fat reduction or any area that has sore or aching muscles due to exertion or exercising.

It is very important in order to get the maximum benefit from a massage to drink plenty of water after the massage. This will enable your body to flush out the toxins that the massage has loosened up. The easier it is for the body to eliminate these toxins the better you will feel and the more fat you will lose.

Physically Masking
Back Fat

Sometimes no matter how hard we try we might not be able to produce the look that we want or lose the fat in certain stubborn places on our body. Some of us are blessed with the body we want while others of us struggle each and every day with problem areas that never seem to get the way we want them to get. When we find ourselves at that point in time, sometimes the best thing to do is look for solutions elsewhere.

There might be a situation where you need to look better fast and will not have the luxury of time to lose the fat naturally. During these times we might have to take matters into our own hands and instead of trying to lose the fat instead we should try and mask it. Fortunately, there are a few ways we can easily accomplish this.

Wear Loose Clothing

If you suffer from love handles, "muffin top" or bra bulge, then you can wear looser fitting clothes so the fat is not as noticeable. Tight clothes will tend to be more form fitting and therefore show off every excess bit of fat on your back and everywhere else. So instead, pick out an outfit that is loose so no one will be the wiser when it comes to your back fat!

Where Different Undergarments

Try and stay away from undergarments that have tight elastic or narrow straps. The tighter the elastic the more it will push against the fat and be noticeable. For undergarments with straps, wear models with wider straps so they will not "dig in" to your skins and make the fat noticeable. Your aim should be for no visible indications of any undergarments.

There are also "control" type undergarments designed to mask fat and smooth out the lines of your body and hide the fat. If you can find an appropriate garment that does a good job that could be an easy "fix" for your problem.

Loosen Up the Belt!

If you can, loosen your belt a notch or two so the belt is not squeezing you at the waist and causing that muffin top or love handles. Keep it only as tight as it needs to be to keep your pants up.

Watch Your Posture!

Do not slouch! Instead walk proud and confident. Keep straight and do not hunch over which might draw attention to your back and other areas. Not only will this help hide the back fat but also do wonders for your body language as well making you look more confident and in control.

Conclusion

I hope by the time you get to this page that you have more than a few ideas on how you are going to tackle getting rid of your back fat. While there are several ways you can go about it, we want to go over a couple of important things before we turn you lose on the treadmill and the dining table!

First of all, remember that there is no easy weight loss magic pill or product that is going to help you change your appearance without some effort on your part. Save your time and money and just do it right from the beginning.

Second, whatever you do, do it healthy. Your health is a lot more important than a little muffin top or love handles. You should always lose fat and weight in a responsible and healthy manner so you don't create any additional health problems along the way.

Check with your doctor or medical care giver before starting any fat or weight loss program.

They can guide you and help you create a program that will not only get you to your goal but enable you to achieve your goals in a healthy and responsible manner.

Last, but certainly not least, do this because YOU want to and never to please anyone else. This is your body and you should control how you look and how you feel. So unless there are medical or health reasons for losing weight or reducing fat content, do it for the right reasons. You need to be you and do what is right for you and not because someone else tells you to.

So good luck and here's to the "New You"!

Part Two:

Weight and Fat Loss Tools

Weight Loss Do's

1)   Do eat low calorie foods like fruits and vegetables

2)   Do eat regularly scheduled meals and snacks. Do not skip meals.

3)   Do get regular aerobic exercise

4)   Do make your doctor part of your weight loss plan

5)   Do make sure you are healthy enough for diet and exercise

6)   Do try to lose weight for YOU, not because someone else wants you to.

7)   Do moderate your efforts and diet.

8)   Do everything in a healthy and responsible fashion

9)   Do drink water to stay hydrated.

10)   Do ask others for their support and assistance

11)   Do your best to stick with your weight loss plan

12)   Do be honest with yourself while setting goals and making choices

13)   Do take time to celebrate success and achieving your goals

14)   Do take time to remind yourself of the benefits of losing weight

15)   Do stay focused and motivated no matter what it takes.

16)   Do adjust or change goals as conditions require

17)   Do your best. No one can ask for anything more.

18)   Do lose weight at a responsible and healthy rate.

19)   Do monitor your progress frequently to catch problems early

20)   Do address and resolve behavioral issues that lead you to eat.

Weight Loss Don'ts!

1)   Don't Skip Meals
2)   Don't cut back on water
3)   Don't reduce your calories per day to starvation levels
4)   Don't do more exercise than you can safely do
5)   Don't try and lose weight too fast!
6)   Don't try to do everything all at once
7)   Don't skip steps in your plan
8)   Don't resort to dangerous fad diets or diet products
9)   Don't do anything that you feel is unhealthy
10)   Don't ignore doctors' advice or warnings
11)   NEVER purge yourself after eating! NEVER!
12)   Don't do anything to excess. Always use moderation
13)   Don't get discouraged. Practice patience and discipline
14)   Don't expect things to change without a behavior change.

15) Don't ignore aches and pains or hurt when exercising.

16) Don't exercise the same body parts every day. Let them heal.

17) Don't forget to stretch before exercising and cool down after.

18) Don't try and do it alone. Ask for help and support from others.

19) Don't be stubborn! Adjust goals and plans as things change

20) Don't Give Up!!!!!!!

Negative Calorie Foods

Eat More & Lose More!

Here is an interesting concept. Negative calorie foods are foods that require more energy and calories to digest than they actually have in them. What that means is that you burn more calories during the processing and digesting of those foods than they had in the food itself.

Here is a list of some negative calorie foods:

Fruits

apple
Cranberries
Grapefruit
lemon
mango
orange
pineapple
raspberries
strawberries
tangerine

Vegetables

asparagus
beets
broccoli
cabbage (green)
carrot
cauliflower
celery
Chile
peppers (hot)
cucumber
dandelion
endive
garden cress
garlic
green beans
lettuce
onion
papaya
radishes
spinach
turnip

We are not saying to create an entire diet made up of these fruits and vegetable but it certainly couldn't hurt to use some of these items in your meals and snacks. Not only will you fill yourself up, but they are essentially "free" calories when used in moderation.

If you want a more complete listing of these foods, or some more information on negative calorie foods, just go online and do a search under "negative calorie foods".

Just make sure they are part of a balanced and nutritious diet and do not over do it!

For more information on how to lose back fat and other How-To Publication on a wide variety or topics, please visit our website at:

http://www.26ways.com

www.ingramcontent.com/pod-product-compliance
Lightning Source LLC
Chambersburg PA
CBHW070817290526
45795CB00002B/746